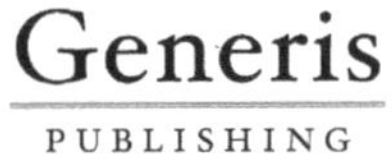
Generis
PUBLISHING

AF582376

Cardiac-Specific Markers in Patients with Acute Myocardial Infarction

Dadabayeva Nailya Akramovna
Mahmudova Munira Safiyevna
Kim Andrey Rudolfovich

Title: **Cardiac-Specific Markers in Patients with Acute Myocardial Infarction**

ISBN: 979-8-89248-720-7

Author: Dadabayeva Nailya Akramovna, Mahmudova Munira Safiyevna,Kim Andrey Rudolfovich

Cover image: www.pixabay.com

Publisher: Generis Publishing
Online orders: www.generis-publishing.com
Contact email: info@generis-publishing.com

Cardiac-specific markers in patients with acute myocardial infarction

Dadabayeva Nailya Akramovna

PhD, Associate Professor

Mahmudova Munira Safiyevna

PhD, Senior Lecturer, Tashkent Medical Academy
maxmudovamunira44@gmail.com

Kim Andrey Rudolfovich

Doctoral Student, Republican Specialized Scientific and Practical

Medical Center of Cardiology. Tashkent, Uzbekistan
kimandrey266@gmail.com

Table of contents

LIST OF ABBREVIATIONS

WHO -World Health Organization

CVD - Cardiovascular diseases

IHD - ischemic heart disease

DM - Diabetes mellitus

AH -Arterial hypertension

PCI - Percutaneous coronary intervention

PICS - Postinfarction cardiosclerosis

CHF - Chronic heart failure

FC -functional class

AF-Atrial fibrillation

GFR - Glomerular filtration rate

HR - Heart rate

LVH - left ventricular hypertrophy

BMI - Body Mass Index

ECG - Electrocardiography

ECHO -Echocardiography

AMI - Acute myocardial infarction

MI - Myocardial infarction

ESR - Erythrocyte sedimentation rate

LDH - Lactate Dehydrogenase

ALT - Alanine aminotransferase

AST - Aspartate aminotransferase

CPK- Creatine Phosphokinase

T - Troponin

H-FABP - Heart-type fatty acid-binding protein

ARF - Acute renal failure

Annotation

The diagnosis of acute myocardial infarction in the first hours after its development is important for the development of proper management tactics for patients.

An important place in this regard is given to biochemical research methods, in particular, the study of serum troponin and myoglobin levels, as one of the methods of early diagnosis. Troponin is a highly specific cardiac marker in AMI, 8-12 hours after the onset of anginal pain. In international practice, the so-called 99th percentile is used, the excess of which makes it possible to diagnose AMI. Normally, there is so little myoglobin in the blood that it is not detected by laboratory methods. When skeletal muscles or myocardium are damaged, myoglobin enters the bloodstream in large quantities. (Plebani M1, Zaninotto M). Myoglobin begins to rise 1-2 hours after myocardial injury, reaches its peak after 8-12 hours and usually returns to normal by the end of the day. (/A.F. Kinle. -M, 2002) Troponin is the "gold standard" in determining a heart attack, but the advantage of myoglobin is that it reacts as early as possible, thereby allowing a faster diagnosis. Normal values of myoglobin range from 0 to 80 ng/ml, with damage to the heart muscle, the content increases 4-10 times (Titov, V.N. / V. N. Titov, T. I. Kotkina, E. I. Volkova //Klin. lab. Diagnostics, 1993).

Detecting troponin and myoglobin, allows for early diagnosis of acute MI, to determine the severity, treatment tactics and rehabilitation of patients.

Introduction

According to WHO, cardiovascular diseases occupy the first place in terms of the frequency and number of deaths. According to WHO estimates, 17.9 million people died from CVD in 2016, accounting for 31% of all deaths worldwide. 85% of these deaths occurred as a result of myocardial infarction and stroke. With the development of new modern technologies (analyzers), the diagnosis of AMI at an early stage is becoming increasingly possible. In addition to changes in the ECG, there are a number of cardiac specific markers: troponin I, myoglobin, CK-MB, LDH, ALT/AST and the relatively new H-FABP, which help to diagnose or exclude AMI, due to their high sensitivity and specificity. Some of them are detected in the blood even with minor lesions of the heart muscle. This is crucial in further treatment tactics, prognosis of the course and rehabilitation of patients.

Myoglobin is one of the highly sensitive cardiac markers that is diagnosed in the blood in the first hours after the onset of anginal attacks. Myoglobin, as an oxygen-binding enzyme, is highly sensitive to oxygen deficiency. Under normal conditions, myoglobin does not enter the bloodstream. In medicine, myoglobin is used to determine the diagnosis of AMI by the appearance of a specific "cardiac" isotype. Due to the high toxicity and size of the molecule, myoglobin is considered dangerous to be in the bloodstream, as it can contribute to blockage of the renal tubules and the development of acute renal failure. In this regard, high myoglobin levels may be prognostically important for the outcome of the disease, as they are the cause of the development of acute kidney injury and later become the cause of death.

Goal

To study the sensitivity and dependence of troponin and myoglobin on the clinical course in patients with acute myocardial infarction.

Chapter I. Literature review

Cardiovascular diseases (CVD) are the leading cause of death worldwide: for no other reason do so many people die every year. Among CVD, the priority place belongs to acute myocardial infarction (AMI), an urgent clinical condition caused by necrosis of a section of the heart muscle as a result of impaired blood supply. By 2030, it is projected that about 23.6 million people will die, mainly from heart disease and stroke. Cardiomarkers play an important role in diagnosis, being able to diagnose early and carry out thrombolytic therapy in the first hours.

The main clinical manifestation of MI is pain syndrome. The pain is characterized by a prolonged attack of angina pectoris (lasting more than 20-30 minutes), poorly relieved by nitroglycerin. Physical examination, as a rule, provides little information confirming the diagnosis of MI, except for the weakening of heart tones and the appearance of additional tones (III or IV). Sometimes it is possible to identify transient cardiac arrhythmias and various changes in blood pressure. Thus, the analysis of clinical data in most cases suggests the development of acute coronary syndrome in a patient, however, laboratory and instrumental studies are necessary in order to confirm or deny the presence of MI.

1.1. Laboratory diagnostics of AMI

Laboratory confirmation of acute MI is based on the identification of: 1) non-specific indicators of tissue necrosis and inflammatory response of the myocardium; 2) hyperfermentemia and 3) an increase in the content of myoglobin and troponins in the blood. The nonspecific reaction of the body to the occurrence of acute MI is primarily associated with the breakdown of muscle fibers, absorption of protein breakdown products into the blood and local aseptic inflammation of the heart muscle, developing mainly in the periinfarction zone. The main non-specific clinical and laboratory signs reflecting these processes are:

1. An increase in body temperature (from subfebrile numbers to 38.5–39 ° C).

2. Leukocytosis, usually not exceeding 12-15 · 109 / L.

3. Aneosinophilia.

4. A small shift of the blood leukocyte formula to the left.

5. Increase in ESR.

High hopes have been pinned on the determination of serum levels of enzymes contained in cardiomyocytes since an increase in the activity of aspartate aminotransferase (AST) in the blood of patients with AMI was discovered in the mid-50s of the XX century. Over the past 30-40 years, biochemical markers have been firmly included in the diagnostic arsenal. Back in 1979. The World Health Organization (WHO) has included biochemical markers in the criteria for the diagnosis of AMI, along with typical ECG changes and clinical symptoms.

By the end of the 80s of the XX century, a fairly well-defined group of biochemical indicators used for the diagnosis of AMI had been formed. Currently, a large number of enzymes are known to be contained in the myocardium: lactate dehydrogenase (LDH), aspartate aminotransferase (AST), Gamma-glutamyl transpeptidase (GGT), aldolase, pyruvate kinase, etc.

However, their "cardiospecificity" is very conditional. In world practice, they have lost their importance, giving way to more specific markers of myocardial necrosis. These include the MB fraction of CK, myoglobin, troponins T and I. Markers such as light and heavy chains of myosin, carbonic anhydrase III, myeloperoxidase, matrix metalloproteinase, placental growth factor, ischemia-modified albumin, H-FABP, pregnancy-associated plasma protein A (PAPP-A), glycogen phosphorylase BB are under study.Currently known cardiac markers can be divided into groups based on their intracellular localization in the cardiomyocyte:

1. Cytosolic - myoglobin; CK; CK-MB; LDH; glycogen phosphorylase BB; protein binding fatty acids.

2. Cytosolic plus structural - troponins T and I.

3. Structural - actin, light and heavy chains of myosin.

The greater the mass of necrotized myocardium, the greater the enzyme output from cardiomyocytes. At the same time, both the level of enzyme content in myocardial tissues and the dynamics of its increase in the blood are important. Since the increase in various cardiac specific enzymes does not occur at the same time, it can be said that the "leaching" of enzymes from the affected myocardium into the blood is not the only mechanism for their release in myocardial infarction. The change in the concentration of markers in the blood during myocardial necrosis is determined by intracellular localization, molecular weight, tertiary structure, half-life, and the state of local blood and lymph circulation. Unbound cytosolic proteins enter the circulatory system more quickly, and their appearance depends on the reperfusion of the infarction zone. The entry of structural proteins into the blood depends on the activation of proteolytic enzymes that destroy the contractile apparatus of the cell. This process takes a long time, and such markers are detected in the blood much later than the appearance of clinical symptoms and remain elevated for a long time. The change in the concentration of these biomarkers does not depend on the reperfusion of the necrosis zone. The kinetics of markers having both a cytosolic pool and a pool of structurally related proteins are similar to cytosolic ones in the early stages, and structurally related proteins in the later stages. Thus, the appearance of a cytosolic troponin T pool strictly depends on the reperfusion of the infarction zone, while the release of a structurally related pool does not depend on reperfusion. Taking into account these features, it is customary to divide cardiac markers of necrosis into early and late.

The very concept of "myocardial necrosis" according to modern views is based on an increase in the level of cardiac specific biomarkers. In 2000, a joint group of experts from ACC/ANA and ESC proposed a new definition of myocardial infarction based on the determination of troponin levels. In accordance with the latest recommendations for the revision of definitions in 2007. The diagnosis of AMI can be established on the basis of an increase and subsequent decrease in the levels of cardiac biomarkers, preferably troponin T and I, exceeding the value of 99 percentile for the upper limit of the norm, in combination with at least one of the following signs of myocardial ischemia: 1) a clinical symptom of ischemia; 2) ischemic changes on the ECG; 3) pathological Q waves on the ECG; 4) a decrease in viable myocardium or the appearance of regional contractility disorders of the heart wall according to imaging methods. This definition has been called "universal". Cardiac troponins I and T, which are characterized by high sensitivity and specificity, are currently accepted as the "gold standard" for the diagnosis of myocardial necrosis. However, it should be noted that an increase in the concentration of cardiac markers reflects only the very fact of the presence of myocardial necrosis, but does not give an idea of its causes. Therefore, in the absence of clinical symptoms of ischemia, it is necessary to search for other possible causes, such as acute pulmonary embolism, chronic heart and kidney failure, myocarditis, and aortic dissection.

In 2011, the official recommendations of the European Society of Cardiology on the management of patients with ACS without ST segment elevation included for the first time the use of highly sensitive troponins (hs-cTn) for the diagnosis of AMI, the diagnostic value of which is higher than traditional tests. Their diagnostic capabilities are currently being studied.

The main provisions of the biochemical diagnosis of MI can be formulated as follows:

1. Biomarkers of myocardial necrosis should be determined in all patients with ACS symptoms and should be used in combination with clinical symptoms and ECG data.

2. It is preferable to determine the highly sensitive troponin T or I.

3. If it is impossible to determine troponins, the best alternative is CK-MB.

4. Total CK, AST and LDH should not be used as cardiac markers due to their low specificity.

5. It is advisable to jointly define "early" (Myoglobin) and "late" (Troponins) markers.

6. Diagnostic information content depends on the timing of MI and the frequency of determination in dynamics.

7. An increase in troponin levels in the absence of clinical manifestations of myocardial ischemia requires the search for other causes of myocardial damage.

Thus, biochemical markers are an integral part of the modern diagnostic strategy for ACS. They allow not only to establish a diagnosis, but also to determine the degree of risk in patients with ACS. Based on the determination of their concentration, important decisions are made about the need for hospitalization of the patient and the degree of aggressiveness of the therapeutic approach.

The practical application of well-known cardiac markers in the early diagnosis of AMI has a number of significant disadvantages. Therefore, the need for an ideal marker of myocardial necrosis, which would be highly sensitive and informative in the early stages of AMI, remains high. An ideal biochemical marker should have the highest specificity and sensitivity to myocardial necrosis, reach a diagnostically significant level in the blood within a short time after the onset of MI symptoms, and this level should be maintained for many days.

The criteria of a cardiac marker.

- Cardiospecificity. The biomarker should not be present in extracardial tissues and should be detected in the blood under any physiological and pathological conditions, that is, it should have absolute cardiospecificity.

- Specificity. The level of the marker should differ in reversible (ischemia) and irreversible (necrosis) myocardial damage.

- Sensitivity. The biomarker should normally be absent in the blood and increase only with myocardial necrosis.

-The kinetics of the marker in the blood. The marker should rise in the blood after myocardial necrosis as early as possible for early diagnosis.

-The marker should circulate in the blood from several hours to several days after myocardial injury and have a sufficiently long half-life for the possibility of late verification of the diagnosis.

-The level of the marker in the blood should correlate with the size of myocardial necrosis

- The removal of the marker from the body should be predictable and not depend on comorbid conditions.

-The ability to quantify and qualitatively measure it in the blood using reliable, fast, affordable, accurate and inexpensive methods.

-The diagnostic value of the marker should be confirmed in clinical studies.

-The marker should have a predictive value.

-The definition of the marker should influence the treatment tactics.

The currently used cardiac markers do not meet these criteria. Therefore, it is recommended that they use two markers in parallel for diagnosis - "early" and "late". The concentration of the "early" marker in AMI reaches a diagnostically significant level in the first hours of the disease, and the "late" one only after 69 hours, but the latter should have a higher specificity for myocardial necrosis.

The closest to the ideal marker is troponin (T and I). However, the use of cardiac troponins has a number of disadvantages. A relatively late increase in the level of troponins in the blood limits their use in the first hours of the disease. In addition, an increase in their level can occur not only in AMI, but also in other pathological conditions. Thus, the problem of early biochemical diagnosis of AMI has not yet been solved. Due to the disadvantages of commonly used and well-studied markers, the search for an optimal marker of myocardial necrosis, more sensitive and specific, continues.

1.2. Transaminases

Aspartate aminotransferase (AST) is a test for the diagnosis of AMI at the first aid level in small clinical diagnostic laboratories. In typical cases of acute MI, AST activity becomes higher 6-12 hours after the appearance of anginal pain, reaches a maximum after 18-36 hours and returns to normal by 3-4 days of the disease. When an increase in activity is associated with concomitant pathological processes (chronic hepatitis, pancreatitis, etc.), it is necessary to determine the ratio of AST to alanine aminotransferase (ALT). In AMI, the ratio of AST/ALT is greater than 1.33, and in liver diseases, the ratio is less than 1.33. But by itself, this increase cannot indicate that the patient has AMI. Additional laboratory testing of other enzymes is necessary, which can reliably confirm the preliminary diagnosis.

Creatine kinase (CK) is found in skeletal muscles, myocardium, brain and thyroid gland. Therefore, an increase in the activity of this enzyme in blood serum is possible not only in acute MI, but also in a number of clinical situations (with heavy physical exertion, after surgery, in patients with muscular dystrophy, myopathy, strokes, hypothyroidism, after coronary angiography, etc.). With the development of a heart attack, an increase in the activity of CK in the blood is usually noted 6-8 hours after the attack. By the end of the first day, the enzyme level is 3-20 times higher than normal, and after 3-4 days from the onset of the disease it returns to its initial values. An increase in the activity of CK in the blood is detected in almost all patients with AMI. It is necessary to determine the activity of CK upon admission and then with an interval of 8-12 hours, in cases of recurrence of pain, it is determined immediately and 12-24 hours after an angina attack. Due to the fact that an increase in CK activity is noted in skeletal muscle injuries, including seizures and prolonged immobilization, non-coronary myocardial diseases, surgical operations, and pulmonary embolism, an additional criteria for diagnosing MI with increased CK and AST activity is the value of the CK/AST ratio. If this ratio is greater than 14, 20 and 25, respectively, with CK activity up to 1200 IU/l and more (norm 38/174 IU/l), then with 95% confidence we can talk about the presence of AMI in patients. An increase in the activity of the MB fraction of CK, contained mainly in the myocardium, is specific for damage to the heart muscle, primarily for AMI. The MB fraction of CK does not respond to damage to skeletal muscles, brain and thyroid gland. After 3-4 hours from the onset of the attack, the activity of MB-CK begins to increase, reaches a maximum after 10-12 hours, and returns to the initial figures 48 hours after the onset of the anginal attack. The degree of increased activity of CK-MB in the blood generally correlates well with the size of a myocardial infarction: the larger the volume of damage to the heart muscle, the higher the activity of CK-MB.

1.3. Lactate Dehydrogenase

The activity of lactate dehydrogenase (LDH) increases in diseases of the myocardium, liver, shock, congestive circulatory insufficiency, pulmonary embolism, coronary angiography, heavy physical exertion, etc. In acute MI, it increases more slowly than CK and CK-MB and remains elevated for longer. LDH activity increases after 5-6 hours from the onset of a painful attack, after 2-3 days the peak of activity occurs and normalizes on 8-14 days. A repeated increase in LDH activity may indicate both a repeat MI and be a consequence of a secondary lesion of the liver parenchyma, resulting from a decrease in the contractility of the heart muscle.The definition of LDH isoenzymes is more specific. LDH1 isoenzyme is more specific for heart lesions, although it is also present not only in the heart muscle, but also in other organs and tissues, including red blood cells. LDH1 activity in MI increases after 3-4 hours and may remain increased for 10-15 days. The increase in LDH1 has the highest diagnostic significance in the first 16-20 hours of MI, when the total LDH does not exceed the norm [4]. A relative increase in LDH1 activity can also be observed after total LDH has returned to normal. The diagnostic criteria is not only an increase in the activity of isoenzymes, but also a change in the LDH1/LDH2 ratio. In patients with MI, it is 0.76 and higher with a norm of 0.45-0.74. The sensitivity of this indicator as a diagnostic MI test is 40-95%, and the specificity is 85%, which in terms of diagnostic effectiveness is close to the definition of CK-MB [2].

1.4. Gamma glutamyltransferase

Gamma glutamyltransferase (GGT). The dynamics of changes in activity (GGT) characterizes the effectiveness of scarring of the necrotic zone of the myocardium. Normalization of activity by 4-5 weeks indicates the completion of this process, which is a good prognostic sign. At the same time, it is necessary to exclude the possibility of hyperfermentemia of GGT associated with the presence of cholestasis, cirrhosis of the liver, malignant tumors of the liver and pancreas.

Table 1

Time intervals of diagnostic significance of the study of enzyme activity in acute myocardial infarction

№	Name of the enzyme	The beginning of an increase in activity(hours)	Maximum increase in activity(h)	Duration of hyperfermentemia*	The timing of normalization of activity
1	AST	3-12	24-36	72 h	36-72 h
2	ALT	3-12	6-12	12 h	6-12 h
3	LDH(total)	6-12	36-78	1-2 week.	2-3 week.
4	LDH1	6-12	36-72	1-2 week.	2-3 week.
5	LDH2	6-12	36-72	1-2 week.	3 week.
6	CK	6-12	18-24	3-4 days.	4 days.
7	CK-MB	4-6	4-12	24 h	24-48 h

Table 2

Diagnostic sensitivity and specificity of laboratory tests in myocardial infarction

Laboratory test	Sensitivity,%	Specificity,%
Aspartate Aminotransferase	87-89	48-88
Creatine kinase(total)	98-100	57-88
After 4 hours	20	89
After 10 hours	59	83
Creatine Kinase MB	94-100	98-100
After 4 hours	16	87
After 10 hours	53	87
Creatine Kinase MB(mass)	94-100	98-100
After 4 hours	49	94
LDH total	87	88
LDH1	40-90	85
Myoglobin	75-95	70
Troponin T	>98	80
After 4 hours	50	100
After 10 hours	100	100
After 7 days	84	100
Troponin I	>98	95

1.5. Myoglobin

Myoglobin (MG) is a low molecular weight heme-containing protein located in the cytoplasm of cardiomyocytes and muscle tissue cells. Its function is the intracellular transport of oxygen. Myoglobin is excreted from the body by the kidneys. Due to the peculiarities of its kinetics, the myoglobin content in AMI increases in blood serum within 2 hours from the onset of anginal pain, reaches its peak after 4-6 hours and returns to normal values after 24-48 hours.

Myoglobin is currently a recognized early marker of myocardial necrosis and is recommended for use in patients with AMI (class 1, evidence level B). Numerous studies have proven its high diagnostic sensitivity in the first 6 hours of AMI. However, factors such as the identity of the amino acid sequence of myoglobin molecules contained in skeletal muscles and in the myocardium, the high content of myoglobin in skeletal muscles, the dependence of concentration on kidney function explain its low specificity for myocardial necrosis and limit its use for the diagnosis of AMI. An increase in the concentration of myoglobin in the blood can be caused by diseases and injuries of skeletal muscles, heavy physical exertion, alcoholism, and kidney failure.

It is clear that myocardial necrosis causes an increase in the level of not only enzymes into the blood, but also other contents of myocytes, in particular myoglobin. This is the basis for the diagnostic test – detecting the myoglobin content in the blood, which under normal conditions does not exceed 85 ng / ml, and in case of myocardial infarction can rise to 1000-1500 ng / ml or more. The diagnostic value of the myoglobin level is reached within 4 hours after the pain attack. The high concentration lasts only a few hours. The small molecular weight allows myoglobin to easily pass through the glomerular membrane of the kidneys, which leads to a rapid drop in plasma concentration. If you do not repeat the analysis, you can skip the peak of its concentration. Therefore, normal results of determining the level of myoglobin in the blood do not exclude acute myocardial infarction. In this case, the diagnostic value of determining myoglobin is significantly inferior to measuring the activity of CK, and even more so CK-MB.

Table 3

Sensitivity and specificity of biomarkers of acute myocardial infarction by hours

Biomarker	**Sensitivity,%**			**Specificity,%**
	3 hours	6 hours	12 hours	
Myoglobin	69 [48-86]	100 [87-100]	100 [87-100]	46 [33-60]
TnI	54 [33-73]	81 [61-93]	100 [87-100]	90 [80-96]
TnT	51 [26-70]	78 [58-89]	100 [82-96]	89 [78-95]
CK	31 [14-52]	54 [33-73]	88 [70-97]	66 [52-78]
CK-MB mass	46 [27-67]	88 [70-97]	100 [87-100]	78 [66-88]

Preference for measuring the concentration of myoglobin can be given only if patients are admitted to the hospital less than 6-8 hours after the attack. It can be concluded that it is impractical to measure the concentration of myoglobin in urine, since it has been shown that with a high concentration capacity of the kidneys, the concentration in urine can be high in absolutely healthy people. According to Shalaev S.V., Petrik E.S., it was shown that myoglobin in the first 3 hours is the most specific with a sensitivity of 69%, surpassing CK-MB and CK, which had 46 and 31%.

1.6. Troponins

With the advent of highly sensitive tests and the subsequent detection of troponins in all healthy people, the attention of researchers is directed to studying the ways of troponin release from intact myocardial cells. The most studied mechanisms of troponin release from the myocardium of healthy individuals are: processes of regeneration and renewal of myocardial cells, apoptosis of cardiomyocytes, release of troponin in membrane vesicles, release of fragments of proteolytic degradation of troponins, increased permeability of cardiomyocyte cell membranes, small-scale (subclinical) necrosis of myocardial cells. It is worth noting that some of these pathways play an important role in pathological processes.

Using the labeled radioisotope 14C integrated into the DNA of cardiomyocytes, evidence of myocardial cell renewal is presented, the intensity of which decreases with age. So, at the age of 25, about 1% of cardiomyocytes per year are divided in humans, they gradually decrease and at the age of 75 they amount to 0.45%; It is calculated that about half of cardiomyocytes are renewed over a lifetime, which indicates the presence of a weak regenerative process. Circadian variation in concentrations is typical for most cells. The greatest severity of daily fluctuations is observed in the levels of hormonal indicators and metabolic substances, on which these hormones exert their influence. Several studies have shown the presence of circadian fluctuations in troponin concentration, on the basis of which it was believed that they should be taken into account when setting the values of the 99th percentile, and the delta of the increase in troponin concentration in patients taken to the emergency department with suspected acute myocardial infarction. This need is due to the fact that the early algorithms used diagnostics of myocardial ischemia are based on taking into account very low concentrations of troponins and even their minor changes can lead to a false positive or false negative interpretation of the analysis results. It has recently been shown that troponin T, determined by the highly sensitive method (Roche Diagnostics), has a daily fluctuation in concentrations: maximum in the morning (8:00), then its decrease is observed and reaches minimum values by about 20:00, after which a smooth increase begins again, which again reaches a maximum in the morning.

The average values in the morning and evening are 16.2 ng/l and 12.1 ng/l. It is believed that the daily rhythm of troponin release (according to highly sensitive methods) should be taken into account for screening purposes. In some cases, circadian features of troponins can affect diagnostic accuracy for AMI. So, van der Linden N.

(2016) estimated the daily fluctuation of hs-TnT and hs-TnI concentrations in an elderly patient with severe chronic renal insufficiency (GFR =14 ml/min). The concentration of cardiac troponin T in blood serum has been chronically elevated for many years in the absence of acute coronary events, which highlights the role of the kidneys in troponin elimination. Troponins are a universal structure of protein nature for striated muscles, localized on thin myofilaments of the contractile apparatus of the myocardiocyte. The troponin complex consists of three components: troponin C is designed for binding calcium, troponin T is for binding tropomyosin, and troponin I is for inhibiting these processes.

In case of myocardial damage, after 4-6 hours due to the development of irreversible necrotic changes, troponin enters the peripheral bloodstream, the peak concentration is reached in the first 12-24 hours from the moment of acute MI. Troponin T and troponin I exist in myocardial-specific isoforms, which determines their absolute cardiospecificity. For troponins, the ratio of concentration inside muscle cells to concentration in blood plasma is much higher than for enzymes and myoglobin, which makes these proteins highly sensitive markers of myocardial damage. Cardiac isoforms of troponin retain their presence in peripheral blood for a long time: troponin I is determined for 5-7 days (0-0.5 ng/ml), troponin T is determined up to 14 days (0-0.1 ng/ml). It is advisable to conduct a study of troponin I during the examination of patients, both early and late after the manifestation of clinical symptoms. Even a slight increase in troponin levels indicates an additional risk for the patient, since there is a clear correlation between the level of troponin increase in the blood and the size of the myocardial injury zone. This test is useful in deciding on the choice of management tactics for patients with acute coronary syndrome, including patients with unstable angina pectoris. In the normal state of the cardiovascular system, troponin should not be detected in the peripheral bloodstream. Its appearance is an alarming signal of necrotic damage to myocardial tissue. In acute coronary syndrome, elevated troponin I levels are regarded as a sign of myocardial ischemia due to platelet activation and aggregation leading to necrosis. An increase in the concentration of troponin I in patients with unstable angina indicates an unfavorable prognosis and risk of developing AMI in the next 4-8 weeks.

Table 4

Dynamics of TnT, CK-MB and MG in the blood serum of patients with coronary heart disease

Studied indicator	Stages of study					Donors (n-30)
	In admission	1 hour after operation	3 hours after operation	6 hours after operation	9 hours after operation	
TnT	0,009± 0,0002	0,64 ± 0,09	0,37 ± 0,011*	0,27± 0,03*	0,009 ± 0,0002	0,009 ± 0,00002
CK-MB	2,56± 0,22	21,4±3,2	2,6± 0,37*	1,71 ± 0,12	1,04± 0,07	1.84± 0.2
MG	37,5±4,2	347,1 ± 44,2	152,5± 23,2*	67,7± 7,2*	35,8± 9,4	32,1 ±3,8

Note: n- is the number of examined patients and donors; statistically significant difference between indicators: * - p <0.001 of the first day and the following.

1.7. Features of various cardiac markers

K.R.Karibaev, D.I.Makhanov, E.S.Maidyrov, B.S.Seidualieva, in a retrospective analysis of 154 medical histories diagnosed with AMI, in the first hours there was an increase in AST in 47.3% of ALT in 14.2% of patients. At the same time, Troponin T turned out to be positive in the first hours in 70% of cases, while Troponin I was positive in only 52.6%. After 6 hours, with repeated measurement of troponins, their diagnostically significant level reached 90%. The latter may be due to the fact that most of the troponins are located in the contractile apparatus of myocytes and a small part of about 7% is in the cytosol, and therefore, with initial damage, it is cytosolic troponins that are released and only after some time from the contractile apparatus. Transaminases did not undergo significant changes in the future. In conclusion, the authors came to the following conclusion: Troponin has an undeniable advantage over transaminases. Troponin has shown itself to be a highly sensitive marker in AMI.

According to the study, it was determined that the laboratory diagnostic priority of Troponin does not reduce the effectiveness of increasing other cardiac markers, and is the best for diagnosing the CK-MB fraction. Myoglobin remains relevant for the earliest diagnosis of AMI. Smolyaninov, A.B. Clinical laboratory and functional diagnostics of internal diseases / A.B.Smolyaninov. – St. Petersburg: SpetsLit, 2009. – 143 S. Staroverov, I.I. Troponins in cardiology /I.I. Staroverov, A.A. Korotkova, V.N. Titov // Cardiology. Scientific and practical journal. - 2002. – No. 4.– p. 122.

A.M. Kelli and others (2014) in their study concluded that in patients with hs-cTnT levels below 0.5 ng/L (Siemens) and the absence of ischemic changes on the ECG within two hours of the onset of anginal pain, the diagnosis of AMI can be excluded. At the same time, the specificity of the study was 100%, and the negative predictive value was 95% [Kelly A.M., Klim Sh. Does undetectable troponin I at presentation using a contemporary sensitive test rule out myocardial infarction?A cohort study. EmergMed J. 2014. No. 32. pp. 760-763.]

Similar results were obtained in a study by W.E. Carlton and others 2015, where 960 patients were observed. As a result of this work, it can be said that troponins, in the absence of changes in the ECG, can exclude AMI with a probability of almost 100 percent.

In addition, the study by M.R. Shamsiev and co-authors, which compared the sensitivity of CK-MB and troponin I in the diagnosis of AMI with and without a Q wave, showed the high sensitivity of troponin I in the diagnosis of AMI, compared with CK-MB, and its relationship with mortality in Q positive AMI. In addition, the ineffectiveness of troponin I in the diagnosis of the transition of unstable angina pectoris to AMI of any localization was shown, "Bullyuten so RAMS 2003, page 43".

Numerous authors show in their research the high sensitivity and effectiveness of Troponin I in diagnosis, M.N. Mitz and co-authors, (Bulletin of the State Chelyabinsk University 2015, No. 21, pp. 123-126.), which investigated early cardiac markers (troponin, myoglobin CK-MB) in unstable angina pectoris and AMI. The result of the above study was the ineffectiveness of all three markers in unstable angina pectoris as a diagnostic marker. In all three cases, a significant advantage in the diagnosis of AMI by these cardiomarkers was shown in men. When evaluating these cardiac markers in AMI, they proved to be effective and highly sensitive, the first of which was myoglobin up to 6 hours, troponin I from 12 hours, and 12 or more hours of CK-MB.

Troponin I is considered the gold standard in the diagnosis of AMI among cardiac markers, the specificity of which is 95-98%. However, in recent decades, they have begun to put forward a greater specificity of Troponin T in the diagnosis of AMI, the specificity of which, according to various authors, is from 98-100%. One of such studies is I.N. Fedotova and coauthors in which an increase of more than 0.3ng/ml meant myocardial necrosis, and in the case of an increase above this level by more than 3 times, the development of a myocardial infarction. According to the results of the data, we can talk about the effectiveness of troponin I, and its increase even with small-focal AMI, compared with other markers.

As mentioned above, the CK-MB fraction is also a criteria for the diagnosis of AMI in the presence of anginal pain, the relationship of ECG data and others.

Studies by Glatz J. in 1994 showed that H-FABP is highly specific for myocardial damage and its concentration reaches a diagnostically significant level in the blood serum of an AMI patient within 2-3 hours after the onset of the disease. The clearance of H-FABP is similar to that of myoglobin.

Since H-FABP is excreted from the organism mainly by the kidneys, therefore it was determined in the urine of patients with myocardial infarction earlier than 2 hours after the onset of pain, and by the 36th hour its excretion from necrotized myocardium stopped. In addition, an increase in the level of this marker was observed in various rhythm disturbances, this is due to the fact that damage or dysfunction of the cardiomyocyte membrane occurs.

According to a study by R.M. Kalichenko (team of authors, 2013), which studied the use of the express test for H-FNumerous authors show in their research the high sensitivity and effectiveness of Troponin I in diagnosis, M.N. Mitz and co-authors, (Bulletin of the State Chelyabinsk University 2015, No. 21, pp. 123-126.), which investigated early cardiomarkers (troponin, myoglobin CK-MB) in unstable angina pectoris and AMI. The result of the above study was the ineffectiveness of all three markers in unstable angina pectoris as a diagnostic marker. In all three cases, a significant advantage in the diagnosis of AMI by these cardiomarkers was shown in men. When evaluating these cardiomarkers in AMI, they proved to be effective and highly sensitive, the first of which was myoglobin up to 6 hours, troponin I from 12 hours, and 12 or more hours of CK-MB.

Troponin I is considered the gold standard in the diagnosis of AMI among cardiomarkers, the specificity of which is 95-98%. However, in recent decades, they have begun to put forward a greater specificity of Troponin T in the diagnosis of AMI, the specificity of which, according to various authors, is from 98-100%. One of such studies is I.N. Fedotova and coauthors in which an increase of more than 0.3ng/ml meant myocardial necrosis, and in the case of an increase above this level by more than 3 times, the development of a mycordial infarction. According to the results of the data, we can talk about the effectiveness of troponin I, and its increase even with small-focal AMI, compared with other markers.

As mentioned above, the CK-MB fraction is also a criteria for the diagnosis of AMI in the presence of anginal pain, the relationship of ECG data and others.

Studies by Glatz J. in 1994 showed that H-FABP is highly specific for myocardial damage and its concentration reaches a diagnostically significant level in the blood serum of an AMI patient within 2-3 hours after the onset of the disease. The clearance of H-FABP is similar to that of myoglobin.

Since H-FABP is excreted from the organism mainly by the kidneys, therefore it was determined in the urine of patients with myocardial infarction earlier than 2 hours after the onset of pain, and by the 36th hour its excretion from necrotized myocardium stopped. In addition, an increase in the level of this marker was observed in various rhythm disturbances, this is due to the fact that damage or dysfunction of the cardiomyocyte membrane occurs.

According to a study by R.M. Kalichenko (team of authors, 2013), which studied the use of the express test for H-FABP in patients with ACS, it was revealed that the level of H-FABP begins to rise in the first hours (79 out of 100 patients were diagnosed with AMI). The specificity in the first hours of H-FABP was 84.8% (67 out of 79 patients), and 98.7% (78 patients) after 6 hours. We can safely talk about its high early sensitivity.

In addition, R. Kalichenko and co-authors also analyzed the comparative predictive significance of cardiac markers, as a result of which H-FABP, along with troponins, demonstrated high rates, especially in the first 2-6 hours.ABP in patients with ACS, it was revealed that the level of H-FABP begins to rise in the first hours (79 out of 100 patients were diagnosed with AMI). The specificity in the first hours of H-FABP was 84.8% (67 out of 79 patients), and 98.7% (78 patients) after 6 hours. We can safely talk about its high early sensitivity.

In addition, R. Kalichenko and co-authors also analyzed the comparative predictive significance of cardiac markers, as a result of which H-FABP, along with troponins, demonstrated high rates, especially in the first 2-6 hours.

Table 6

Dynamics by the hours of cardiac markers of AMI

Marker	2 hours		6 hours		24 hours	
	PPV	NPV	PPV	NPV	PPV	NPV
Troponin I	100	28.8	100	77.8	100	100
Myoglobin	96.3	41.3	97.4	86.4	-	-
CK-MB	100	25.6	100	60	100	77.8
H-FABP	100	63.6	100	95.5	100	86.4

The main result of the work of Kalichenko R and co-authors was that H-FABP can become differentially and diagnostically significant in the diagnosis of AMI and unstable angina pectoris, and exclude AMI at early stages.

According to a study by A.S. Salnikov and co-authors (Bulletin of the Russian Academy of Medical Sciences Volume 12,2012), which, referring to various authoritative publications and articles, shows in its article the dominance of H-FABP over myoglobin and more specific and sensitive compared to the latter (specificity reached 93.1%). In 535 cases, it was H-FABP that was positive and only in 355 Troponin I, the sensitivity of which was 73.8% and 46.7%. However, sensitivity was determined in 325 patients in whom Troponin I was H-FABP. The latter is the case to exclude the diagnosis if there is a suspicion of AMI.

Table 7

Sensitivity and specificity of H-FABP and troponin in patients with AMI

Time before emerge of symptoms(hours)	Sensitivity(%)		Specificity(%)	
	H-FABP	Troponin I	H-FABP	Troponin I
1-3	65.8	37.9	87	95.9
3-6	84	52.2	95.9	96.9
6-12	70.6	52	94.3	99

After the study of Kokorin G.A. together with co-authors in 2017, conducting a subanalysis of the research work, in which 592 patients participated, according to the results of laboratory data, it was determined that the rapid test of H-FABP was positive in 57.8%, while Troponin was only 44.3%. The conclusions of this work confirmed that H-FABP turned out to be more sensitive and more accurate in the first 6 hours compared to troponin I, which may indicate its ability to determine AMI at the earliest possible time.

Conclusions

Due to the fact that AMI is one of the most common diseases that cause the death of patients, its early diagnosis is the main key in the treatment and prognosis of the course of the disease. To present days, many studies have been conducted on cardiomarkers capable of diagnosing AMI. Troponin I has become the "gold standard" in the diagnosis of AMI. Myoglobin – allows you to clarify the diagnosis of AMI in the first hours after the onset of anginous pain. A large number of scientific works show how important myoglobin is in the early diagnosis of AMI in order to predict the right tactics in treatment, because besides the fact that it is a specific enzyme, its presence in the blood carries a great danger to human life due to blockage of the renal tubules and as a result of acute renal failure.

CHAPTER II. RESEARCH MATERIALS AND METHODS

95 AMI patients aged 40-75 years were examined, among them 51 men (53.4%) and 44 women (46.6%).

General characteristics of patients

Table-1

Distribution of AMI patients depending on the age and gender of patients

AMI	45-59 ages n=54		60 and over ages n=41		Total
	Males	Females	Males	Females	
with Q n =40	13 (24.07%)	8(14.81%)	9 (47.3%)	10(24.3%)	40
without Q n=55	18 (33.3%)	15(27.78%)	11(50%)	11(26.83%)	55
Overall	31 (57,4%)	23 (42,6%)	20(97.3%)	21 (51,13%)	95

AMI was more common in men, but the difference became zero with age. In middle-aged women, AMI is more common than in young women.

The patients underwent clinical laboratory diagnostic and instrumental examination.

1 – Clinical

Inquiry (Complaints and anamnesis)

Examination (general examination and physical examinations of the cardiovascular, respiratory, digestive, urinary and endocrine systems)

2- Laboratory diagnostic

General blood test, general urine test

Biochemical blood tests (ALT, AST, lipids, glucose, urea, creatinine, coagulogram)

3-Cardiomarkers (transaminases, troponin I, myogobin)

Transaminases, troponin I and myoglobin were determined by immunological method using a Rosche analyzer (Germany). Troponin I can be present in small amounts in the blood, therefore, for a more accurate diagnosis, the concept of 99-percentile troponin has been introduced, which corresponds to the upper limit of reference values.

In general, the level corresponding to the 99th percentile is specific for various diagnostic kits of different manufacturers; its values are -

– for the hscTnI Singulex Erenna test - 8.0 ng/l; -

-for Abbott ARCHITECT's hscTnI test – 12 ng/L; -

-for Roche's hscTnT test - 14 ng/L;

- for the hscTnI PATHFAST Mitsubishi test – 20 ng/L;

- for the hsTnI ADVIA Centaur Siemens test - 40 ng/l.

Determination of the level of myoglobin in the blood serum

It was carried out in the first hours after admission and was determined by Rosche (Germany) immunological method on an analyzer. Currently, myoglobin is the earliest biological marker of myocardial necrosis. Its small molecular weight (17,800) causes faster penetration into the blood compared to enzymes such as CK (MW = 80,000) or LDH (MW = 130,000). Myoglobin appears in the peripheral blood 2-3 hours after the onset of pain and reaches a pathological level 3-6 hours earlier than CPK-MB. The peak concentration of myoglobin is observed after 6-9 hours, and the peak concentration of cardiac enzymes is observed only after 12-19 hours.

Reference values range from 25ng/ml to 70ng/ml

4 – Instrumental

-ECG (in 12 standard leads)

-Echocardiography

Statistical processing of research materials

Data storage and primary processing were carried out in the Microsoft Excel 2010 database using the Statistica 10 program.

CHAPTER III. THE RESULTS OF OUR OWN RESEARCH

3.1. The results of clinical data

AMI was accompanied by severe pain in 93%, while pain-free AMI was in 7% of patients and was accompanied by palpitations, shortness of breath, weakness and fear. The development of AMI in most patients occurred against the background of increased blood pressure in 67.4% from 140 to 200 mmHg, and in 22.05% of patients who had various complications, there was a decrease in blood pressure below 80-60 mmHg. Tachycardia was observed in 88%, bradycardia in 3.4%. Complications were more common in patients with AMI with a Q wave (92%).

Auscultatively, all patients had muffled tones and 20 (21.05%) had various rhythm disturbances (extrasystole, atrial fibrillation, paroxysmal tachycardia).

The most common clinical symptom was severe chest pain, which is associated with a high myocardial oxygen demand.

Table-2

The relationship of anginal pain with blood pressure figures

84 patients with typical anginal pain		11 patients without anginal pain	
Elevation of BP	**Decrease in BP**	**Elevation of BP**	**Decrease in BP**
38 (45,2%)	16 (19,0%)	6(54,5%)	3(27,2%)

Pain syndrome in 38 (45.2%) patients was accompanied by increased blood pressure up to 190/110mmHg and in 16 (19%) blood pressure decreased below 80/50mmHg. With pain-free AMI, the predominance of the number of patients with high blood pressure over low was also observed. In more than half of the patients, 49 (51.5%) had tachycardia up to 120 beats/min. and 7 (7.3%) had bradycardia, with a decrease in heart rate to 54 beats/min.

Table-3

Clinical symptoms depending on the location of AMI

Location	Clinical symptoms					
	Pain N=84 (88,4%)	Dyspnea N=11 (11,5%)	HR >90/min N=49 (51,5%)	HR <60/min N=7 (7,3%)	BP>140 mmHg N=52 54,7%)	BP<80 mmHg N=31 (32,6%)
Anterior wall	12 (14.28%)	1 (9%)	5 (10.2%)	1 (14.28%)	9 (17.3%)	1 (3.2%)
Anterior septal area	22 (26.2%)	2 (18.18%)	12 (24.4%)	2 (28.5%)	11 (21.1%)	6 (19.35%)
Anterior apical area	15 (17.8%)	2 (18.18%)	10 (20%)	1(14.28%)	13 (25%)	6 (19.35%)
Diffuse AMI	15 (17.8%)	3 (27.27%)	12 (24.4%)		14 (27%)	4 (12.9%)
Lateral wall	4 (4.7%)		3 (6.1%)	1 (14.28%)		3 (9.6%)
Posterior wall	16 (19%)	3 (27.27%)	7 (14.2%)	2 (28.5%)	5 (9.6%)	11 (35.4%)

The most common clinical symptom was severe pain, which was more often observed in antero-septal MI (26.2%) and in lateral localization (4.7%). An increase in blood pressure was more common with diffuse MI (27%).

Tachycardia was observed in 49 (58.3%) patients, and depended on the localization, so with anteroposterior, anterior-apical and diffuse AMI, it was more common. The rarest symptom is bradycardia, which was registered in 7 (8.3%) patients.

43 (55.8%) patients developed life-threatening complications: 24 (25.2%) of them had acute left ventricular failure, 7 (16.2%) had atrial fibrillation, ventricular extrasystoles had 4 (9.3%), 4 (9.3%) had supraventricular tachycardia, cardiogenic shock in 3 (6.9%), 1 (2.3%) has ventricular tachycardia.

Table-4

Number of patients developed life-threatening complications after AMI

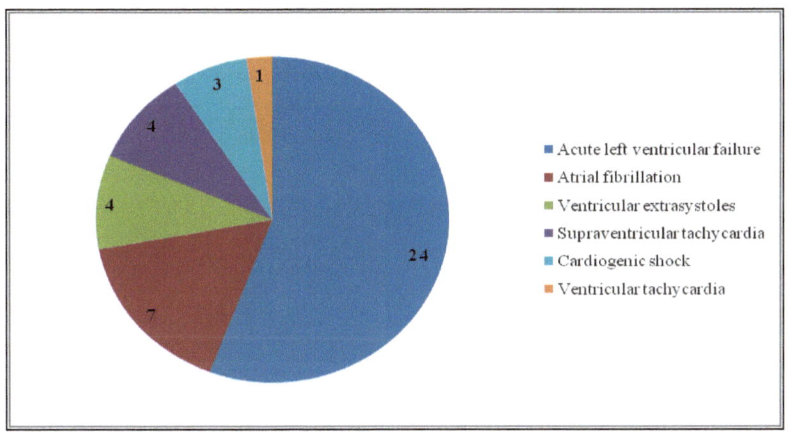

Acute left ventricular failure was the most common complication of AMI, and ventricular tachycardia was the rarest.

3.2. Results of laboratory and instrumental research

The level of cardiomarkers in patients with AMI with a Q wave at various clinical parameters was more often increased in the presence of pain, decreased blood pressure and the development of complications. Transaminases increased in 23% of patients with pain, TnI in 82%, and myoglobin in 86%. The maximum level was observed with a decrease in blood pressure. The severity of the clinical course, namely complications, contributed to an increase in the level of transaminases, which were recorded in 30% of patients. Myoglobin and TnI had a stable tendency to increase by more than 80%.

Table-5

Increased levels of transaminases, troponin I and myoglobin in patients with AMI with a Q wave, depending on various clinical parameters

AMI with Q wave	Pain		AP		HR		Complications
	present	absent	AP> 140 mmHg	AP< 80 mmHg	>90	<60	
Transaminases	23%	7,3%	12%	21%	12%	14%	30%
TnI	82%	80%	76%	87%	75%	60%	84%
Myoglobin	86%	75%	82%	88%	78%	80%	80%

Table-6

Increased levels of transaminases, troponin I and myoglobin in patients with AMI without a Q wave, depending on various clinical parameters

AMI without Q wave	Pain		AP		HR		Complications
	present	absent	AP> 140 mmHg	AP< 80 mmHg	>90	<60	
Transaminases	5.2%	2.7%	6.5%	9.3%	8.1%	9.3%	22,5%
TnI	80%	81%	84%	82%	82%	74%	82%
Myoglobin	89%	79%	86%	88%	76%	80%	80%

In the presence of pain, an increase in ThI and myoglobin in comparison with transaminases was observed in a larger number of patients. In the pain-free form of AMI, similar results were obtained. In the latter case, the diagnosis of AMI was made based on ECG data and increased cardiac markers.

With a decrease in blood pressure, all enzymes were elevated in a large number of patients with a change in heart rate, transaminases were inferior in sensitivity to myoglobin and troponin I. Complications were accompanied by an increase in transaminase in a large number of patients. Myoglobin and TnI in both AMI with and without a Q wave showed high sensitivity and specificity, surpassing transaminases.

At the same time, in pain syndrome, myoglobin was maximal in 89% of patients, TnI increased in 80%, while transaminases increased only in 5.2% of patients. With bradycardia, TnI was positive in 74% of patients and only 76% of patients with tachycardia had increased myoglobin. Transaminases increased in 2.7% of patients with pain-free AMI. The minimum of myoglobin accounted for tachycardia in 76%, and in 2.7% of patients transaminases increased with pain-free AMI. The maximum increase in transaminases was noted with the development of complications in 22.5%, when myoglobin. In the presence of pain increased TnI and myoglobin in comparison with transaminases was observed in a larger number of patients. In the pain-free form of AMI, similar results were obtained. In the latter case, the diagnosis of AMI was made according to ECG data and increased cardiac-specific markers.

Transaminases, depending on different clinical parameters in AMI, showed low sensitivity, increasing in AMI with a Q wave, and reaching a maximum at the anterior septum localization. In AMI without a Q wave, transaminases increased more often in the antero-septum and apical regions. If in AMI with a Q wave, transaminases increased as much as possible in patients with localization on the anterior septum wall, then with the same localization in AMI without a Q wave, it was observed in a minimum number of patients (8%).

Table-7

Sensitivity of Transaminases in patients with AMI

		Location					
		Anterior wall	**Anterior septal**	**Anterior apical**	**Diffuse AMI**	**Lateral wall**	**Posterior wall**
Transaminases	**AMI with Q wave**		**33%**	**16.7%**	**20%**		**23%**
	AMI without Q wave		**8%**	**25%**		**16,7%**	**25%**

Transaminases increased more often in patients with AMI with a Q wave, and they also showed no sensitivity when localized on the anterior wall.

Troponin I showed its high sensitivity, increasing in more than 50% of patients with each localization of AMI, reaching a maximum in patients with a Q wave in the antero-apical region and lateral wall (100% of patients), somewhat less often on the anterior wall of the left ventricle. A similar trend was observed in AMI without a Q wave.

Table-8

Sensitivity of Troponin I in patients with AMI

		Location					
		Anterior wall	**Anterior septal**	**Anterior apical**	**Diffuse AMI**	**Lateral wall**	**Posterior wall**
Troponin I	**AMI with Q wave**	**50%**	**66.7%**	**100%**	75%	100	92,2%
	AMI without Q wave	**50%**	**66,7%**	**80%**	**66,7%**	**50%**	**75%**

In AMI with a Q wave, an increase in the level of TnI was observed more often than in AMI without Q, reaching a maximum in the antero-apical region and side wall. An increase in TnI was more often noted with localization in the anterior apical region both with AMI with Q and without the Q wave.

Myoglobin showed high sensitivity and was positive on average in 85.4% of patients.

Table-9

Myoglobin sensitivity in patients with AMI

		Location					
		Anterior wall	**Anterior septal**	**Anterior apical**	**Diffuse AMI**	**Lateral wall**	**Posterior wall**
Myoglobin	**AMI with Q wave**	66,7%	100%	100%	75%	100%	80%
	AMI with out Q wave	100	75%	100%	100	66,7%	66,7%

Regardless of the size of the AMI, Myoglobin had an equally high sensitivity. With different localization, myoglobin indices were different in AMI with a Q wave. The level of myoglobin increased in 66.7% and 75%, respectively, on the anterior wall and common AMI, and a maximum in the anterior-septal and anterior-apical and lateral walls in 100% of patients.

Myoglobin in AMI without a Q wave with localization on the posterior and lateral walls increased only in 66.7%, and in 75% of patients in the antero-apical region. Other localizations of AMI showed a higher result: myoglobin increased 100%. At the same time, regardless of the type of AMI with localization in the anteroposterior region, myoglobin levels increased in all patients. When AMI was localized on the back and side walls with AMI with Q, the lowest level of sensitivity was recorded, while in other areas the maximum indicator was noted. At the same time, myoglobin increased more often in AMI with Q wave, which was accompanied by massive necrosis.

When comparing cardiac markers with each other, troponin occupied a central place, due to its high sensitivity and specificity. Transaminases showed little effect, increasing only in 25% of patients, at most as in AMI with and without a Q wave. The sensitivity of myoglobin did not depend on the degree of necrosis, increasing in the blood in more than 80% of patients. Troponins and myoglobin, according to many studies, have shown high sensitivity in AMI. At the same time, myoglobin was significantly superior in AMI without a Q wave. On the LV lateral wall, myoglobin and troponin increased in a small number of patients in 66.7% and 50%, respectively, while transaminases did not increase at all.

Table-10

Comparative sensitivity of transaminases, troponin I and myoglobin in patients with AMI.

Location	with Q wave			Without Q wave		
	Transaminases	TnI	myoglobin	Transaminases	TnI	myoglobin
Anterior wall		50%	66,7%		50%	100%
Anterior septal	33%	66.7 %	100%	8%	66,7 %	75%
Anterior apical	16,7%	100 %	100%	25%	80%	100%
Diffuse AMI	20%	75%	75%	16.7%	66.7 %	100%
Lateral wall	-	100 %	100%	-	50%	66.7%
Posterior wall	23%	92,3 %	80%	25%	75%	66.7%
Total	15.45%	80.1 %	87%	12.45%	64.73 %	84.3%

In AMI with a Q–wave, the sensitivity of troponin I and myoglobin is relatively the same, and in AMI without a Q-wave, myoglobin was much superior to troponin I.

Figure-1

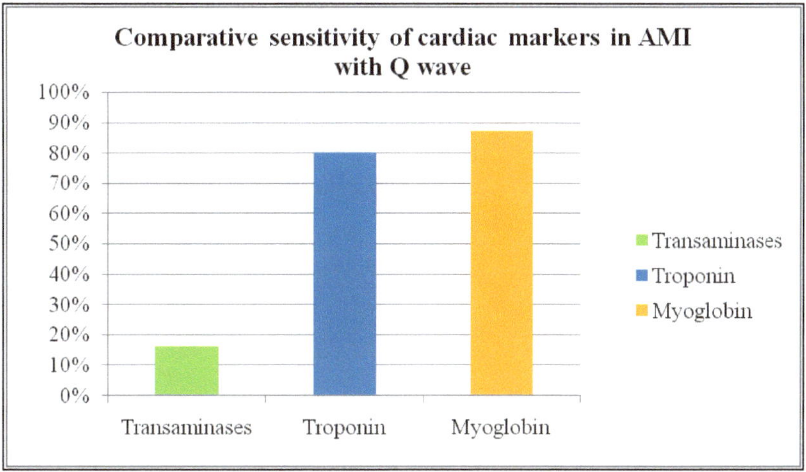

In AMI with Q, the sensitivity of troponin and myoglobin is almost the same and exceeds the transaminase indices.

Figure-2

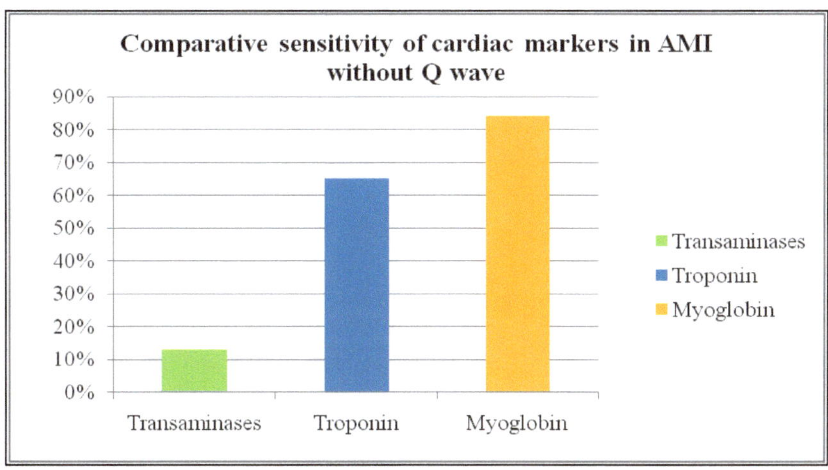

In AMI without Q, myoglobin dominates over other markers.Complications determined the severity of the clinical course of AMI, the most common of which was acute left ventricular failure, in which myoglobin and troponin increased in 85% and 83% of patients, respectively. The highest rate was observed in cardiogenic shock. Troponin and myoglobin increased in 100% of patients, and transaminases in 66.7%.

In case of rhythm disturbances (ventricular tachycardia, atrial fibrillation, extrasystole), transaminases did not increase. Myoglobin did not show its sensitivity either, with ventricular tachycardia and extrasystoles. In atrial fibrillation, Myoglobin was superior to other cardiac markers and was detected in 100% of patients.

Table-11

Sensitivity of transaminases, troponin and myoglobin in patients with AMI with complications.

Complications	transaminases	Troponin I	Myoglobin
Acute left ventricular failure	54,3%	85%	83,3%
Cardiogenic shock	66,7%	100%	100%
Ventricular tachycardia		100%	
Supraventricular tachycardia	50%	100%	100%
Atrial fibrillation		50%	100%
Ventricular extrasystoles		50%	

In case of complications, TnI showed high sensitivity, confirming the severity of the course of AMI. Transaminases showed the lowest sensitivity.

The analysis of cardiomarkers and general blood analysis showed that Myoglobin in the first hours exceeded all other cardiomarkers and increased in 85.5% of patients, while Troponin I in 74%. Transaminases, leukocytosis and elevated ESR were low and increased in 14%, 15% and 4% of patients, respectively.

Figure-3

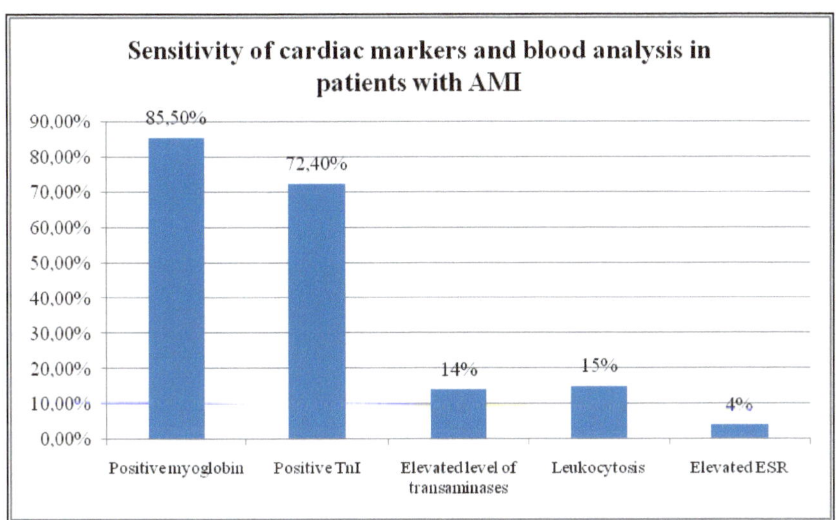

Myoglobin and troponin I showed the highest sensitivity when compared with leukocytosis and elevated ESR.

Conclusion

Among cardiovascular diseases, special attention is paid to AMI, which is the cause of a greater number of deaths among the population. Diagnosis is usually not difficult if there are obvious clinical signs and changes on the ECG. According to numerous authors, AMI occurs with severe pain syndrome. In addition to pain, frequent clinical signs are changes in blood pressure and heart rate. Due to the presence of atypical forms of AMI, as well as the development of a pain-free form of AMI, and sometimes not so pronounced pain syndrome, it can be difficult to diagnose AMI. The absence of obvious focal changes on the ECG also complicates diagnosis. For the correct tactics of treatment of patients, the correct diagnosis plays an important role, therefore, since the middle of the last century, so-called markers of myocardial necrosis have been developed for the diagnosis of AMI, which play an important role in the diagnosis of AMI. Transaminases are considered the first in clinical practice, and then because of the higher sensitivity and specificity of Troponins. According to reputable publications and research, the level of specificity of troponins exceeds 70 percent. According to the latest standards, an increase in troponins in the blood indicates AMI, even in the absence of changes on the ECG. The disadvantage of troponins is their not so rapid appearance in serum, which is sometimes necessary to choose the right tactics. In this regard, in recent decades, there has been interest in another representative – myoglobin. The latter is highly sensitive in the early hours, helping to diagnose AMI at an early stage.

We studied the features of the clinical course of AMI: more than 90% of patients had severe pain syndrome, as well as either an increase in blood pressure of 71% or a decrease of 7.3%. At the same time, troponin and myoglobin levels increased in more than 70% of patients. An increase in the content of transaminases was detected only in ¼ of patients. In case of complications, Troponin and myoglobin also showed high sensitivity, increasing on average in 80-100%. The latter played an important role in the diagnosis of the pain-free form of AMI, where the main clinical symptom was severe shortness of breath.

Determination of the level of transaminases, troponin I and myoglobin, showed low sensitivity of transaminases, and high importance of troponin I, in 74% of patients. High sensitivity of myoglobin was also detected in the early hours, it exceeded the threshold values (maximum 510 ng/ml.) and was determined in 88% of patients. In 2 cases, with continued anginal pain and negative Troponin I, an increase in Myoglobin levels was observed, which further contributed to the choice of management tactics for patients. The results obtained fully reflect the data of scientific research, articles, monographs, and various clinical and diagnostic materials. Thus, Troponin showed its high sensitivity in 74% of patients. Myoglobin in the early hours turned out to be the most informative, while other cardiomarkers are not detected in the blood. Myoglobin exceeded the permissible values by 5-6 times. Transaminases have 8-33% sensitivity. At the same time, cardiomarkers made it possible to diagnose AMI in early and controversial situations, when no changes were detected on the ECG and the clinic was minimal. Thus, cardiomarkers have different sensitivity and their level depends on the clinical manifestations of the size of the necrosis focus and its localization.

1. The most common clinical symptom of AMI was pain in 88.4% of patients, hypertension was somewhat less common in 54.7%, and the rarest clinical sign was bradycardia, which was detected in 7.3% of patients.
2. When compared with clinical symptoms, Troponin I and myoglobin showed greater sensitivity than transaminases.
3. In the first hours of AMI, myoglobin has a higher sensitivity, increasing 5-6 times, to 510 ng/ml (norm 24-72 ng/ ml) than Troponin I and transaminases
4. The sensitivity of Troponin I and myoglobin in AMI with a Q-wave was the same (it was determined in 80% and 87%). However, in AMI without a Q wave, myoglobin was more sensitive (in 81% and 64%).
5. Troponin I and myoglobin increased to the maximum when AMI was localized in the antero-apical region.

Practical recommendations

1. If AMI and ACS are suspected, the duration of which varies within 6 hours, it is recommended to determine myoglobin.
2. If the 6-8 hour threshold is exceeded, the diagnosis of myoglobin is impractical in this case, the level of Troponin should be determined.
3. In the absence of changes on the ECG, but there is a pronounced clinic to confirm the diagnosis of AMI, it is necessary to determine troponin and myoglobin in the blood, depending on the onset of the disease.

List of literature

1.Baturina O. V., Gilyarevsky S. R., Kuzmina I. M., Godkov M.A., Klychnikova E.V. The effectiveness of combined use of biomarker tests for the diagnosis of myocardial infarction in the early stages after the development of its clinical manifestations: the role of a cardiac specific protein binding fatty acids// Rational pharmacotherapy in cardiology. – 2012. – Vol. 8, No. 3. – pp. 405-414.

2.Burns A.S., Zakharova V.A. The role of the cardiac fraction of the fatty acid binding protein in patients with acute coronary syndrome in the long-term prognosis// Topical issues of modern science: collection of materials. SI Monsieur. scientific and practical conf. In the 2nd part of 2018. -pp. 194-198.

3.Brazhnik V.A., Zateyshchikov D.A. The use of necrosis biomarkers for early diagnosis of myocardial infarction in modern conditions//Cardiology. - 2016. - vol. 56. No. 1. - pp. 93-98.

4.Duplyakov D.V., Chaulin A.M. Mutations of cardiac troponins associated with cardiomyopathies // Cardiology: news, opinions, training. - 2019. - Vol. 7, No. 3. - pp. 8-17.

5.Zalevskaya N.G. Modern methods of laboratory confirmation of myocardial infarction//Current problems of medicine. - 2011. – Vol. 14, No. 10 (105). – Pp.260-267.

6.Zalevskaya N.G. Modern methods of laboratory confirmation of myocardial infarction//Scientific bulletin of Belgorod State University. Series: Medicine. Pharmacy. - 2011. - № 10 (105). - Pp. 260-267.

7.Zalevskaya N.G. Modern methods of laboratory confirmation of myocardial infarction// Current problems of medicine. – 2011. – vol. 14, No. 10 (105). – pp.260-267.

8.Kalinichenko R.M., Kopylov F.Yu. Application of high-quality rapid test for fatty acid binding protein for early diagnosis of myocardial infarction//Cardiology and cardiovascular surgery. - 2011. - vol. 4. No. 6. - pp. 16-20.

9.Mars E.T. Appointment as a cardiovascular researcher for the development of the non-profit sector of the Myocardium in men under 60 years of age//Science of the Russian Military Medical Academy. - 2021. - vol. 40. No. C1-3. - pp. 213-216.

10.Mitz N.M., Zyryanova Y.M., Stashkevich D.S. Features of the use of early cardiac markers in the diagnosis of myocardial infarction//Bulletin of the Chelyabinsk State University. - 2015. - № 21 (376). - Pp. 123-127.
11.Mukhtarov T.A., Skvortsov V.V., Tumarenko A.V., Belyakova E.V. Modern biochemical markers in the diagnosis of myocardial infarction//Medical alphabet. - 2016. - Vol. 2. No. 28 (291). - pp. 37-41
12.About Petyunina.V., Kopitsa N.P., Gileva Ya.V., Peteneva L.L., Titarenko N.V. The role of ct2 in patients with acute myocardial infarction with st segment elevation and//Ukrainian Therapeutic Journal. - 2017. - № 1 (52). - Pp. 48-51.
13.Ryabov V.V., Kirgizova M.A., Markov V.A. The use of an express test for the determination of cardiac fatty acid binding protein in the diagnosis of acute myocardial infarction//Russian Journal of Cardiology. - 2014. - vol. 19. No. 2. - pp. 84-88.
14.Trusheva K.S., Toktarbayeva A.A., Baibolova M.K. Cardiac myosin-binding protein c - improved diagnosis of acute myocardial infarction//Issues of science and education. - 2019. - № 2 (45). - Pp. 88-94.
15.Khamitova A. F., Dozhdev S. S., Zagidullin S. Z., etc. Modern cardiac specific biomarkers in different variants of myocardial infarction // Diary of the Kazan medical school. – 2018. – № 4(22). – Pp. 40-46.
16.Shaulin A.M. Some modern BIM markers of the Middle European level: vysotsky, katanin, PCSK-9 // Regional studies. - 2020. - vol. 10. No. 8. - pp. 20-27.
17.Chaulin A.M., Grigorieva E.V., Nurbaltaeva D.A., Duplyakov D.V. Clinical and diagnostic value of cardiomarkers in human biological fluids // Cardiology. – 2019. - No. 59. – p.65.
18.Chaulin A.M., Dublyakov D.V. PCSK-9: new ideas about the biological and economic role and the possibility of using it as a statesman. -Russian scientist. Part 1 // Cardiology: news, opinion, education. - 2019. - Vol. 7, No. 2. - pp. 45-57.
19.Chaulin A.M., Karsyan L.S., Grigorieva E.V., Nurbaltaeva D.A., Duplyakov D.V. Clinical and diagnostic value of cardiomarkers in human biological fluids // Cardiology. – 2019. - № 59(11). – Pp.66-75.
20.Shumyantseva V.V., Bulko T.V., Sigolaeva L.V., Kuzikov A.V., Archakov A.I. Polymer matrices with molecular memory as affine sorbents for the determination of myoglobin as a cardiomarker of acute myocardial infarction by voltammetry//Journal of Analytical Chemistry. - 2017. - vol. 72. No. 4. - pp. 357-362.

21.Aydin S., Ugur K., Aydin S., Sanin I., Yardim M. Biome markers at the opening of the Micard market: new research. //Market Management for hello, January 2019, January 17;15:1-10.
22.Jay Chen, Zhang V., Wu I.K., Chen H., Zhao J.F. Correlation of acute myocardial infarction complicated by cerebral infarction with insulin resistance, adiponectin and HMGB1 protein. //Euro Turnover Honey Pharmacol. Econ. Sciences May 2019; 23(10): 4425-4431.
23.D Chistyakov.A., Orekhov A.N., Bobryshev Yu.V. Cardiospecific microRNAs in cardiogenesis, heart function and heart pathology (with an emphasis on myocardial infarction). // J Mol Cell Phone Renovation. May 2016; 94:107-121.
24.Danezeh., Montenyana M. Historical approach to the diagnostic biomarkers of acute coronary syndrome.// Ann Transl Med. 2016, May;4(10):194.
25.Han Jay, Ma Jay, Xia N, Song L, Li B, L. Clinical significance of the combined use of CK-MB, MYO, cTnI and NT-trial exposure in the diastolic space of myocardial infarction.// Clinical laboratory. 2017, March 1;63(3):427-433.
26.Jin J., Chen M., Li Yu., Wang Yu., Zhang S., Wang Z., Wang L., Zhu S. Detection of acute myocardial infarction using diffusion-weighted imaging compared with T2-weighted imaging and markers of myocardial necrosis. // The Heart of Texas Institute, 2016, October 1; 43(5):383-391.
27.Kubena P., Spinar Ya., Dastich M., Lokai P., Parzhenitsa Ya. Diagnostic and prognostic biomarkers in acute coronary syndrome. //Evening Lecture Hall, winter 2018;63(12):935-944.
28.Lackner K. J. Laboratory diagnostics of myocardial infarction - troponins and more.// Clinical and Chemical Laboratory, med. 2013, January;51(1):83-9.
29.Lippi J., Servellin J. Immunoassay for cardiospecific troponin: how low is the risk of dose reduction? //Euro 2016, May; 30:e7-e8.
30.Mekel M., Searle J. Copeptin is a marker of acute myocardial infarction. //Curr Atheroscler Rep. 2014, July; 16(7):421.
31.Sabatasso S., Mangin P., Fracasso T., Moretti M., Dokje M., Johnov V. Early markers of myocardial ischemia and sudden cardiac death. //International Law Journal, September 2016; 130(5):1265-80.
32.Streng A.S., van der Linden N.E., Coken D.M., Beckers O., Bowman G.G., Mariman E.M., Mix S.R., Vodig V.K., deb Burd D. Mass spectrometric

identification of medium complexity in most cases, Suffering from acute myocardial infarction.// J Appl Lab Med. 2018 1;2(6): 857-867.

33. Wang P, Yao J, Xie Y, Luo M. Gender-Specific Predictive Markers of Poor Prognosis for Patients with Acute Myocardial Infarction During a 6-Month Follow-up.// J Cardiovasc Transl Res. 2020 Feb;13(1):27-38

34. Agapitov L. I. Early diagnosis of hypertension and prevention of hypertension in children and adolescents based on daily monitoring of blood pressure: Abstract. ... Candidate of Medical Sciences. - M., 2000. – 20 p.

35. Ageev F. T., Ovchinnikov A. G. Diagnosis and treatment of a patient with diastolic heart failure: the role of an isometric load test (clinical observation). Department of Myocardial Diseases and Heart Failure of the A. L. Myasnikov Research Institute of Cardiology of the Russian Academy of Medical Sciences, Moscow // Heart failure. - 2002. - Volume 1, No. 2. – pp. 71-73.

36. Alexandrov A. A., Rozanov V. B. Epidemiology and prevention of high blood pressure in children and adolescents // Russian pediatrician. Journal. - 1998. - No.2. - C. 16-20.

37. Alekseeva A. A., Vakhlakov A. N., Sergeeva E. V., Perov Yu. L., Gasilin V. S., Chorbinskaya S. A., Gribunov Yu. P. Fatal and nonfatal cardiovascular complications in patients with hypertension with long-term follow-up // Cardiology. - 2002. - No. 4. – pp. 23-28.

38. Arabidze G. G., Belousov Yu. B., Varakin Yu. Y. et al. Diagnosis and treatment of arterial hypertension: Methodological recommendations. - M., 1997. - 95 p.

39. Arabidze G. G., Arabidze G. R. Hypertensive crises – classification, diagnosis of complications, treatment // Cardiology. - 1999. - No. 10. – pp. 86-91.

40. Aronov D. M. Prevention of atherosclerosis in people with risk factors and in patients with coronary heart disease // Russian Medical Journal. – 2000.- vol.8.- No.8.- pp.350-358.

41. Arterial hypertension. VII report of the Joint Commission on the Detection and Treatment of Arterial Hypertension with the support of the National Institute of Pathology of Heart, Lungs and Blood // Arterial hypertension. - 2003. – pp. 3-14.

42. Bazina I. B., Bogachev R. S., Kovalev O. I., Ivanteeva T. V., Lifke M. V., Rafeenkova V. S., Shutova E. P. Epidemiological and social aspects of hypertension in young people (according to the results of a survey of the

organized labor collective of Smolensk) // Ter. archive. – 2004. - No.1. – S. 31-33.
43.Baksheev V. I., Kolomoets N. M., Tursunova G. F. Clinical effectiveness of the school of GB patients at the outpatient stage // Ter.archive. 2005. - No. 11. - pp. 49-55.
44.Balkarov I. M., Shonichev D. G., Kozlova V. G., Novikova M. S., Shakhnova E. A., Solovyova O. L. Some approaches to improving the quality of treatment of patients with arterial hypertension (the experience of the "school of a patient with arterial hypertension") // Ter.archive, - 2000. - No. 1. - pp. 47-51.
45.Barth B. Ya. Systolic hypertension in elderly people in the practice of a district therapist // Ter. Arch. – 1994. - No. 10. - pp. 79-81.
46.Batyushin M. M. Prediction of risk factors and family prevention of essential hypertension: Abstract. ... candidate of Medical Sciences. - Rostov n/A, 2000. – 27 p.
47.Baschinsky S. E. Development of clinical practical guidelines from the standpoint of evidence-based medicine. A training manual for doctors and health care organizers. – Moscow:Media Sphere Publishing House, 2004.
48.Belenkov Yu. N., Vorobyov I. A., Galkin V. A., Gogin E. E., Golikov A. P., Elisev O. M., Loginov A. S., Mukhin N. A., Nasonova V. A., Pokrovsky V. I., Silvestov V. P., Sumarokov A.V., Chuchalkin A. G. Polyclinic care. Epidemiology, prevention and treatment of internal diseases // Ter. arch. – 2000. - No.5. – pp. 47-51
49.Belousov Yu.B., Upnitsky A.A., Egorova N.A., Sapunova N.V. Clinical and instrumental study of metoprolol in patients with mild and moderate arterial hypertension in outpatient settings // Cardiology. - 1997. - No. 2. – pp. 14-15.
50.Belyalov F. I. Alcohol and prevention of cardiovascular diseases // Cardiology – 2004. - No. 4. – pp. 78-81.
51.Boitsov S. A., Markov M. A., Hirmanov V. N. Arterial hypertension in residents of St. Petersburg: frequency of occurrence, attitude to prevention and adequacy of therapy // New doctors. vedas – 1997. - No. 1. – pp. 8-10.
52.Bokarev I. N. Arterial hypertension: modern approaches to treatment // Neurole. Journal. - 1998. - No.5. - C. 4-9.
53.Bondarenko B. B. Cardiovascular diseases. Arterial hypertension // Library "Doctor to patient". – St. Petersburg, 2001. – p. 24.

54.Bondar A. I. Arterial hypertension in children and adolescents and the principles of its prevention in an urban polyclinic: Abstract.... Candidate of Medical Sciences. – Kharkov, 1991. – 23 p.
55.Britov A. N. Modern classification of arterial hypertension and its use in secondary prevention // Cardiology. 1996. - No. 8. – pp. 86-93.
56.Britov A. N., Bystrova M. M., Orlov A. A. Stroke prevention is a real task in the practice of cardiologists and therapists. therapy and prevention. - 2002. - №1. - C. 53-60.
57.Britov A. N., Manvelov L. S. Prevention of cerebral circulation disorders in arterial hypertension // Therapist. Arch. - 1997. – Volume 69, No. 1. - C. 38-43.
58.Varakin Yu. Ya. Arterial hypertension and prevention of acute cerebral circulatory disorders // Neurole. Journal. - 1996. - No.3. - C. 11-15.
59.Vereshchagin N. V., Chazov E. I. Arterial hypertension and stroke prevention // A brief guide for doctors. – M., 1996. – p. 31.
60.Vlasov V. V. Introduction to evidence–based medicine. – M.: Media Sphere, 2001. - 147 p.
61.Volkov V. S., Pozdnyakov Yu. M. Treatment and prevention of hypertension. - M.: Anko, 1999. - 192 p.
62.Volkova E. G. Arterial hypertension: A method. recommendations for a lie. technologies of prevention and treatment in adults and children. - Chelyabinsk, 1998. - 52 p.
63.Gavrikov N. A. Hypertension: prevention, diagnosis and treatment // Medicine for you. - Rostov n/A: Phoenix, 2001. - 253 p.
64.Gadzhiev H. E., Gadzhiev A. N. On the early diagnosis of GB // Therapeutic archive – 1997. - No. 4. – pp. 10-12.
65.Gafarov V. V., Pak V. A., Gagulin I. V., Gafarova A.V. Studying on the basis of the WHO MONICA program awareness of their health and attitude to it in men and women aged 25 to 64 years in Novosibirsk // Ter.archive. – 2003. - No.11. – pp. 46-52.
66.Gembitsky E. V. Arterial hypertension // Clinical medicine. - 1997. - No. 1. – pp. 56-60.
67.Glazer M. G., Boyko N. V., Abildinova A. Zh., Sobolev K. E. Risk factors in the Moscow population of patients with hypertension // Russian Journal of Cardiology. – 2002. - No.6. – pp. 1-5.
68.Gogin E. E. Changes in the arterial bed in hypertensive disease and the treatment strategy of patients. // Ter. Archive. – 1999. - No.1. - pp. 64-67.

69.Gogin E. E. Hypertension is the main cause determining cardiovascular morbidity and mortality in the country // Ter. Archive. – 2003. - No.9. - pp. 31-36.
70.Gogin E. E. Prevention and treatment of hypertension - an important condition for medical support of sustainable development of the country // Russian Medical News. - 1998. – Volume 3, No. 2. - pp. 25-31.
71.Gorbachenkov A. A., Pozdnyakov Yu. M., Tsvetkov V. V. Arterial hypertension. - M., 1999. - 50 p.
72.Gorbunov V. M. 24-hour automatic blood pressure monitoring. Recommendations for doctors // Cardiology. - 1997. - No. 6. – pp. 96-104.
73.Gorbunov V. M. The importance of self-measurement of blood pressure in patients with arterial hypertension // Cardiology. - 2002. No. 1. – pp. 58-66.
74.Dementieva N. G. Dynamics of pharmacoepidemiology of antihypertensive drugs in Kursk for six years // Collection of abstracts of the Russian National Congress of Cardiologists (October 8-11, 2002). - St. Petersburg, 2002. – p. 117.
75.Derevyanshin Yu. S. Difficulties in the management of elderly and senile cardiac patients // Siberian Medical Journal. – 1995. - No.1. – pp. 27-29.
76.Dudnevich A. Sh., Clinic and features of the course of GB in the elderly and senile age // materials of the XI scientific conference of therapists "Secondary prevention of internal diseases". – Riga, 1986. – vol. 2. – pp. 19-21.
77.Egorova N. A. Family primary prevention of cardiovascular diseases: approaches to organization and management: Abstract. ... candidate of Medical Sciences. – Novosibirsk, 2000. - p. 30.
78.Zakharov V. N. Early diagnosis and primary prevention of hypertension. – Moscow: Medicine. - 1999. - pp. 52-56.
79.Zelveyan P. A., Buniatyan M. S., Oschepkova E. V., Rogoza A. N., Harutyunyan G. H. The daily rhythm of blood pressure: clinical significance and prognostic value // Cardiology. - 2002. - No. 10. – pp. 55-61.
80.Zueva E. B., Bakieva M. A. Beta-blockers. Clinical pharmacology and principles of therapy from the standpoint of evidence-based medicine. Metoprolol (egilok) and carvedilol (talliton): Methodological recommendations for doctors. - Tashkent, 2006. - p. 88.

81.Ivanov K. I. Epidemiology of coronary heart disease, risk factors and mortality among the male population of Yakutsk: Abstract. diss. ... candidate of Medical Sciences. - M., 1997. – p. 24.
82.Ivanova V. D., Kryukov N. N., Loginova M. V. Controversial issues of secondary prevention of arterial hypertension in primary health care // Collection of abstracts of the Russian National Congress of Cardiologists (October 8-11, 2002). - St. Petersburg, 2002. – p. 155.
83.Study Of The Health Of The Population Of Uzbekistan 2002. Information and Analytical Center of the Ministry of Health of the Republic of Uzbekistan. – Tashkent, 2003. – p. 397
84.Inarokova A.M. Prevention of arterial hypertension among employees of motor transport enterprises: Abstract. ... Candidate of Medical Sciences. - M., 1988. – 23 p.
85.Kanushko A. V., Gidzinskaya I. N. Changes in the function of the left ventricle in elderly patients with GB // Ter. Archive. – 1999. - No.1. - pp. 68-72.
86.Karpov Yu. A. Clinical hypertension: analysis of completed studies 2001-2002. // Cardiology. - 2002. - No. 10. – pp. 62-66.
87.Karpov Yu. A. FLAG – program for achieving target blood pressure levels in the treatment of patients with arterial hypertension with fosinopril // Cardiology. - 2002. - No. 1. – pp. 52-57.
88.Clinical and organizational guidelines for the provision of medical care to patients with hypertension by a general practitioner. - Russia-USA, M., 2001. – 73 p.
89.Clinical guidelines for the diagnosis, treatment and prevention of arterial hypertension in adults in primary health care. - Tashkent, 2005. – 73 p.
90.Klochkov V. A. The use of high-speed analysis of the daily blood pressure profile for the diagnosis and treatment of hypertension // Cardiology. - 1998. - No. 4. – pp. 26-29.
91.Kobalava J. D. ARGUS 2000: the middle of the road // Topical issues of arterial hypertension. The medical publication of the pharmaceutical group. - Servier, 2000. - No. 3. - 11 p.
92.Kobalava J. D. International standards on arterial hypertension: agreed and uncoordinated positions // Cardiology. - 2002. -No. 11. – pp. 78-91.
93.Kobalava J. D., Villevalde S. V. Is patient education a factor that increases the effectiveness of arterial hypertension control? // Cardiology. - 2007. - No. 10. – pp. 75-82.

94.Kobalava Zh. D., Katovskaya Yu. V., Moiseev V. S. Features of morning blood pressure rise in patients with GB with various variants of the circadian rhythm // Cardiology. - 1998. - No.6. – pp. 23-26.
95.Kobalava J. D., Katovskaya Y. V., Starostina E. G., Villevalde S. V., Lukyanova E. A., etc. Problems of doctor-patient interaction and hypertension control in Russia. The main results of the Russian scientific and practical program ARGUS-2 // Cardiology. - 2007. - No.3. – pp. 38-47.
96.Kobalava Zh. D., Katovskaya Yu. V., Shkolnikova B. E. Dynamics of indicators of daily blood pressure monitoring and quality of life in patients with systolic hypertension with arifon monotherapy // Therapeutic archive. – 1998. - No.9. - pp. 67-69.
97.Kobalava Zh. D., Kotovskaya Yu. V., Sklizkova L. A., Moiseev V. S. Treatment and examination of elderly patients with arterial hypertension: doctors' ideas and real practice (according to the Russian scientific and practical program ARGUS) // Ter. archive. - 2002. – Volume 8, No. 5. – pp. 7-12.
98.Kobalava Zh. D., Katovskaya Yu. V., Treshenko S. N., Maksimov V. S. Clinical significance of daily blood pressure monitoring for the choice of treatment tactics for patients with hypertension // Cardiology. - 1997. - No. 9. – pp. 98-104.
99.Kobalava Zh. D., Shkolnikova B. E., Moiseev V. S. Features of quality of life in elderly patients with isolated systolic hypertension // Cardiology. - 1999. - No. 10. – pp. 27-31.
100.Kozlova V. G., Gromov V. L. and others. Kidney damage and hypertension in elderly and senile people // Ter. Archive. – 1996. – Vol. 68, No. 6. – pp. 53-55.
101.Komarov F. I., Bakarev I. N. Arterial hypertension // Clinical medicine. – 1997. No. 6. - pp. 61-66.
102.Konkol K. Y. Secondary prevention of coronary heart disease occurring with the main risk factors of hypertension: Abstract. ... Doctor of Medical Sciences. - M., 1999. – 45 p.
103.Konradi A. O., Soboleva A.V., Maksimova T. A., Polunicheva E. V., Brodskaya I. S., Shlyakhto E. V. Is teaching patients with hypertension a senseless waste of time or a real tool in improving the quality of disease control? Arterial hypertension. - 2002. - No.8. – pp. 6-10.
104.Kuzyeva L. R., Davletshin R. A., A Eliseev. S., V Gaisina. T., Valeev I. G., and Sharipova. A. Arterial hypertension: spread, prevention,

rehabilitation in certain population groups of the Republic of Bashkortostan // Jubilee scientific and practical conference dedicated to the 60th anniversary of the Department of Hospital Therapy of Bashkir State University: Sb. scientific tr. – Ufa, 1997. - pp. 109-111.

105.Kurbanov R. D., Eliseeva M. R. Beta-adrenoblockers in the cardiological practice of a doctor: Methodological recommendations. - T. – 1998. – p. 86.

106.Labeznik L. B., Komisarenko I. A., Milyukova O. M. Arterial hypertension "Treatment of patients of older age groups with mild and moderate arterial hypertension with valsartan" // Cardiology. - 1999. - No. 3. – pp. 23-25.

107.Leonova M. V., Belousov D. Yu. Results of pharmacoepidemiological study of hypertension in Russia (PYTHAGORAS) // Cardiology. - 2003. –

108.Mazur E. S., Gnedov D. F., Bagdanov E. K. Comparative assessment of the effectiveness of antihypertensive therapy by monitoring blood pressure and blood pressure based on the results of single measurements // Klin. med. – 1999. - No. 7. – pp. 50-52.

109.Mazur E. S., Kalyazina V. V. On the clinical significance of blood pressure variability in hypertension // Therapeutic archive. – 1999. - No.1. – pp. 22-25.

110.Makolkin V. I. Nebivolol - a representative of a new generation of beta-blockers // Cardiology. - 2000. - No. 1. – pp. 69-71.

111.Makolkin V. I., Podzolkov V. I., Gilyarov M. Yu. The possibilities of daily blood pressure monitoring in the differential diagnosis of neurocirculatory dystonia and hypertension // Cardiology. - 1997. - No. 6. – pp. 24-28.

112.Mamasoliev N. S., Kamalov I., Garumov A. G. Prevalence of arterial hypertension among men in Andijan // Healthcare of Turkmenistan. - 1988. - No.8. – pp. 43-44.

113.Mammadov M. N., Oganov R. G. Arterial hypertension in the clinical practice of a doctor: a modern strategy for diagnosis and treatment // Medicine. - 2005. - No. 3. – pp. 10-16.

114.Mamutov R. Sh., Mirzaev N. L., Sunnatullaev A. S. Medical examination of persons with hypertension in one of the rural districts of the Tashkent region. Abstracts of the XIX All–Union Congress of Theaters. - M., 1987. – pp. 93-94.

115.Mamasaliev N.S. "Coronary syndrome at prehospital stage: clinics, etiology, pathogenesis, epidemiology, classification and terminology". / N.S. Mamasaliev, A.L. Vertkin, H.H. Tursunov // Uzbekistan in cardiology. No.4. 2018. 59-63 p.
116."Cardiology. General practitioner / R.G. Oganov, I. G. Fomin tahriri ostida - M.: Tibbiyot, 2004. - 852 p.
117.Mamasaliev N.S. "Coronary syndrome at prehospital stage: ECG diagnostics for differential diagnosis" / N.S. Mamasaliev, A.L. Vertkin, H.H. Tursunov // Uzbekistan in cardiology. 2010.No. 4. 63-66 b.
118.Shumyantseva V.V., Bulko T.V., Sigolaeva L.V., Kuzikov A.V., Archakov A.I. Polymer matrices with molecular memory as affine sorbents for the determination of myoglobin as a cardiac marker of acute myocardial infarction by voltammetry//Journal of Analytical Chemistry. - 2017. - vol. 72. No. 4. - pp. 357-362.
119.Aydin S., Ugur K., Aydin S., Sakhin I., Yardim M. Biomarkers in acute myocardial infarction: modern perspectives. //Health Risk Management Vasc. 2019, January 17;15:1-10.
120.Chen J., Zhang V., Wu I.K., Chen H., Zhao J.F. Correlation of acute myocardial infarction complicated by cerebral infarction with insulin resistance, adiponectin and HMGB1. //Eur Rev Med Pharmacol Sci. 2019 May; 23(10):4425-4431.
121.Chistyakov D.A., Orekhov A.N., Bobryshev Yu.V. Cardiac Specific microRNAs in cardiogenesis, heart function and heart pathology (with an emphasis on myocardial infarction). //J Mol Cell Cardiol. May 2016; 94:107-121

www.ingramcontent.com/pod-product-compliance
Lightning Source LLC
LaVergne TN
LVHW021303160826
845679LV00001B/195

* 9 7 9 8 8 9 2 4 8 7 2 0 7 *